Baby Shower For

_____

Date

_____

_____

Copyright © 2020 by Luis Lukesun

All rights reserved. No part of this book may be reproduced without written permission of the copyright owner, except for the use of limited quotations for the purpose of book reviews.

Guest Name

Relationship to Parents

Advice for Parents

Wishes for Baby

Guest Name

Relationship to Parents

Advice for Parents

Wishes for Baby

Guest Name

Relationship to Parents

Advice for Parents

Wishes for Baby

Guest Name

Relationship to Parents

Advice for Parents

Wishes for Baby

Guest Name

Relationship to Parents

Advice for Parents

Wishes for Baby

Guest Name

Relationship to Parents

Advice for Parents

Wishes for Baby

Guest Name

Relationship to Parents

Advice for Parents

Wishes for Baby

Guest Name

Relationship to Parents

Advice for Parents

Wishes for Baby

Guest Name

Relationship to Parents

Advice for Parents

Wishes for Baby

Guest Name

Relationship to Parents

Advice for Parents

Wishes for Baby

Guest Name

Relationship to Parents

Advice for Parents

Wishes for Baby

Guest Name

Relationship to Parents

Advice for Parents

Wishes for Baby

Guest Name

Relationship to Parents

Advice for Parents

Wishes for Baby

Guest Name

Relationship to Parents

Advice for Parents

Wishes for Baby

Guest Name

Relationship to Parents

Advice for Parents

Wishes for Baby

Guest Name

Relationship to Parents

Advice for Parents

Wishes for Baby

Guest Name

Relationship to Parents

Advice for Parents

Wishes for Baby

Guest Name

Relationship to Parents

Advice for Parents

Wishes for Baby

Guest Name

Relationship to Parents

Advice for Parents

Wishes for Baby

Guest Name

Relationship to Parents

Advice for Parents

Wishes for Baby

Guest Name

Relationship to Parents

Advice for Parents

Wishes for Baby

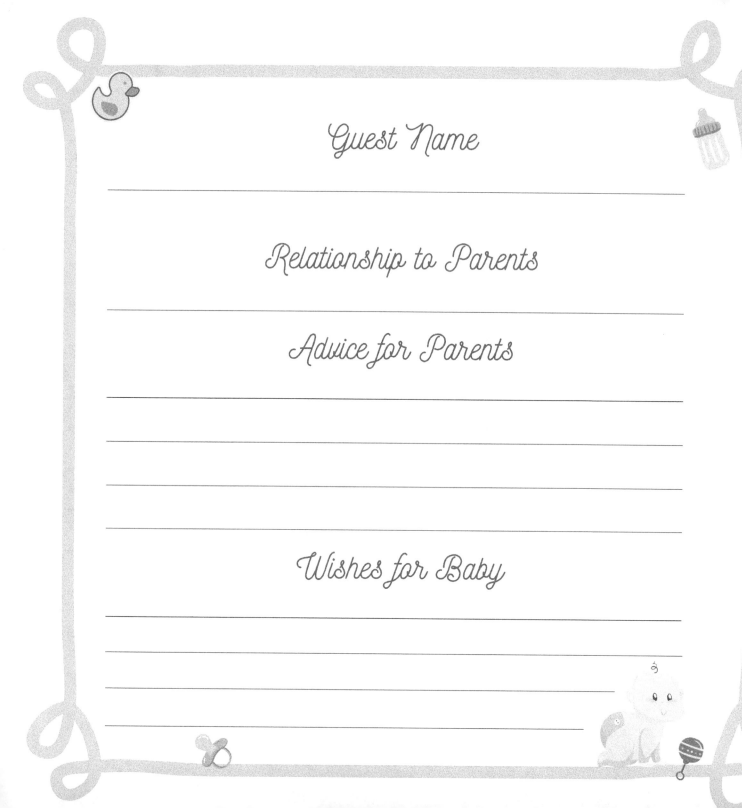

Guest Name

Relationship to Parents

Advice for Parents

Wishes for Baby

Guest Name

Relationship to Parents

Advice for Parents

Wishes for Baby

Guest Name

Relationship to Parents

Advice for Parents

Wishes for Baby

Guest Name

Relationship to Parents

Advice for Parents

Wishes for Baby

Guest Name

Relationship to Parents

Advice for Parents

Wishes for Baby

Guest Name

Relationship to Parents

Advice for Parents

Wishes for Baby

Guest Name

Relationship to Parents

Advice for Parents

Wishes for Baby

Guest Name

Relationship to Parents

Advice for Parents

Wishes for Baby

Guest Name

Relationship to Parents

Advice for Parents

Wishes for Baby

Guest Name

Relationship to Parents

Advice for Parents

Wishes for Baby

Guest Name

Relationship to Parents

Advice for Parents

Wishes for Baby

Guest Name

Relationship to Parents

Advice for Parents

Wishes for Baby

Guest Name

Relationship to Parents

Advice for Parents

Wishes for Baby

Guest Name

Relationship to Parents

Advice for Parents

Wishes for Baby

Guest Name

Relationship to Parents

Advice for Parents

Wishes for Baby

Guest Name

Relationship to Parents

Advice for Parents

Wishes for Baby

Guest Name

Relationship to Parents

Advice for Parents

Wishes for Baby

Guest Name

Relationship to Parents

Advice for Parents

Wishes for Baby

Guest Name

Relationship to Parents

Advice for Parents

Wishes for Baby

Guest Name

_____

Relationship to Parents

_____

Advice for Parents

_____
_____
_____

Wishes for Baby

_____
_____
_____

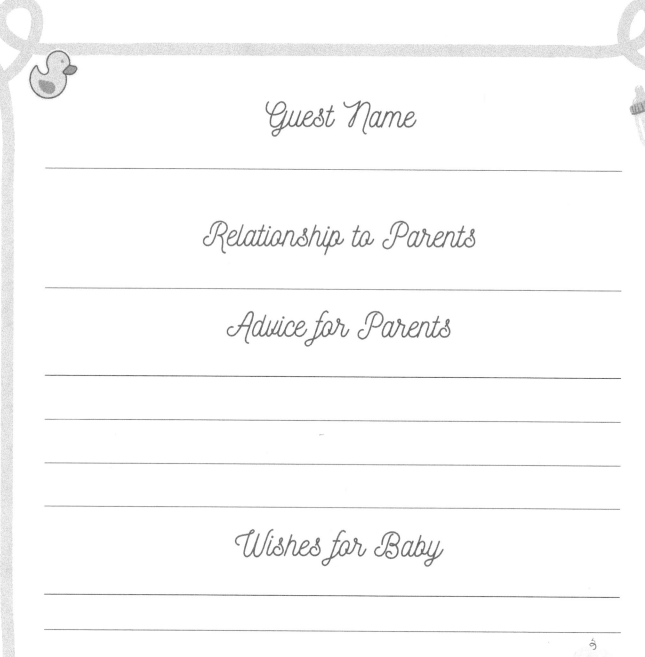
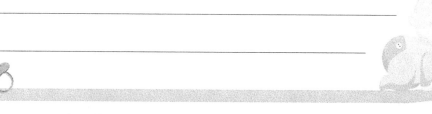

Guest Name

Relationship to Parents

Advice for Parents

Wishes for Baby

Guest Name

Relationship to Parents

Advice for Parents

Wishes for Baby

Guest Name

Relationship to Parents

Advice for Parents

Wishes for Baby

Guest Name

Relationship to Parents

Advice for Parents

Wishes for Baby

Guest Name

Relationship to Parents

Advice for Parents

Wishes for Baby

Guest Name

Relationship to Parents

Advice for Parents

Wishes for Baby

Guest Name

Relationship to Parents

Advice for Parents

Wishes for Baby

Guest Name

Relationship to Parents

Advice for Parents

Wishes for Baby

Guest Name

Relationship to Parents

Advice for Parents

Wishes for Baby

Guest Name

Relationship to Parents

Advice for Parents

Wishes for Baby

Guest Name

Relationship to Parents

Advice for Parents

Wishes for Baby

Guest Name

Relationship to Parents

Advice for Parents

Wishes for Baby

Guest Name

Relationship to Parents

Advice for Parents

Wishes for Baby

Guest Name

Relationship to Parents

Advice for Parents

Wishes for Baby

Guest Name

Relationship to Parents

Advice for Parents

Wishes for Baby

Guest Name

Relationship to Parents

Advice for Parents

Wishes for Baby

Guest Name

Relationship to Parents

Advice for Parents

Wishes for Baby

Guest Name

Relationship to Parents

Advice for Parents

Wishes for Baby

Guest Name

Relationship to Parents

Advice for Parents

Wishes for Baby

Guest Name

Relationship to Parents

Advice for Parents

Wishes for Baby

Guest Name

Relationship to Parents

Advice for Parents

Wishes for Baby

Guest Name

Relationship to Parents

Advice for Parents

Wishes for Baby

Guest Name

Relationship to Parents

Advice for Parents

Wishes for Baby

Guest Name

___

Relationship to Parents

___

Advice for Parents

___

___

___

Wishes for Baby

___

___

___

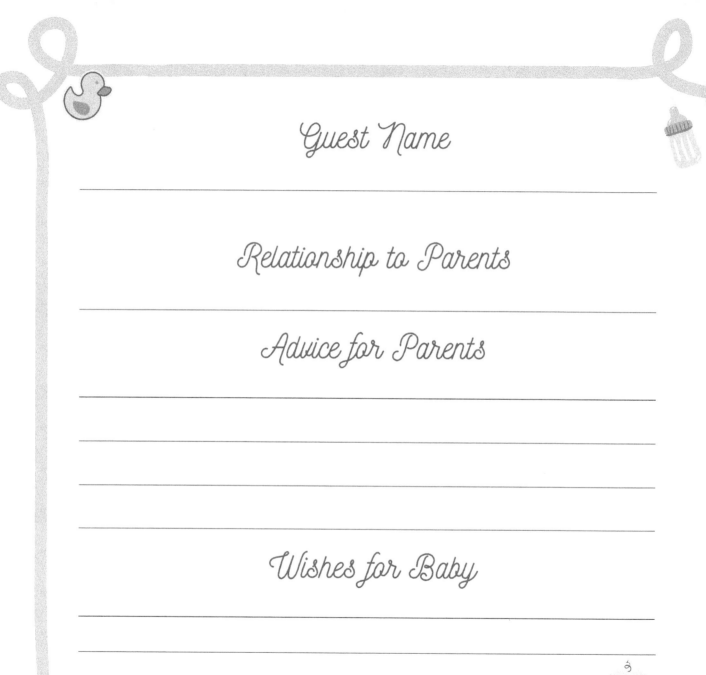

Guest Name

Relationship to Parents

Advice for Parents

Wishes for Baby

Guest Name

Relationship to Parents

Advice for Parents

Wishes for Baby

Guest Name

Relationship to Parents

Advice for Parents

Wishes for Baby

Guest Name

Relationship to Parents

Advice for Parents

Wishes for Baby

Guest Name

Relationship to Parents

Advice for Parents

Wishes for Baby

Guest Name

Relationship to Parents

Advice for Parents

Wishes for Baby

Guest Name

_____

Relationship to Parents

_____

Advice for Parents

_____

_____

_____

Wishes for Baby

_____

_____

_____

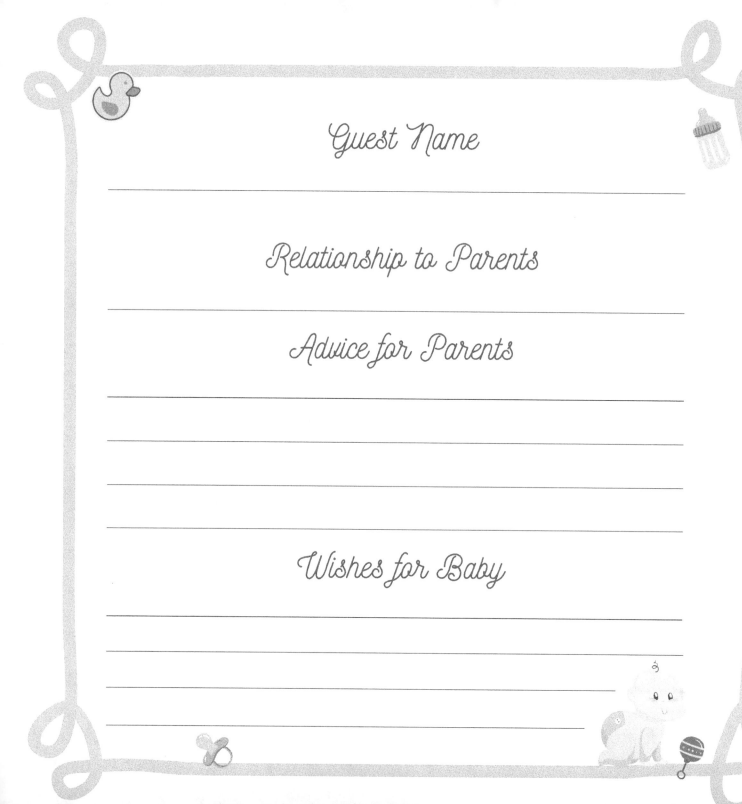

Guest Name

Relationship to Parents

Advice for Parents

Wishes for Baby

Guest Name

Relationship to Parents

Advice for Parents

Wishes for Baby

Guest Name

Relationship to Parents

Advice for Parents

Wishes for Baby

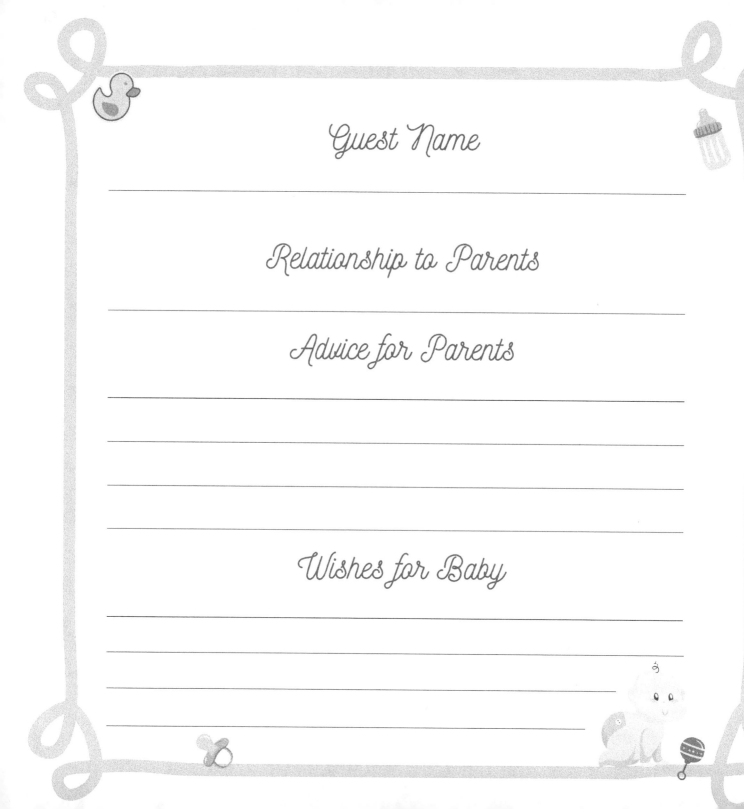

Guest Name

Relationship to Parents

Advice for Parents

Wishes for Baby

Guest Name

Relationship to Parents

Advice for Parents

Wishes for Baby

Guest Name

Relationship to Parents

Advice for Parents

Wishes for Baby

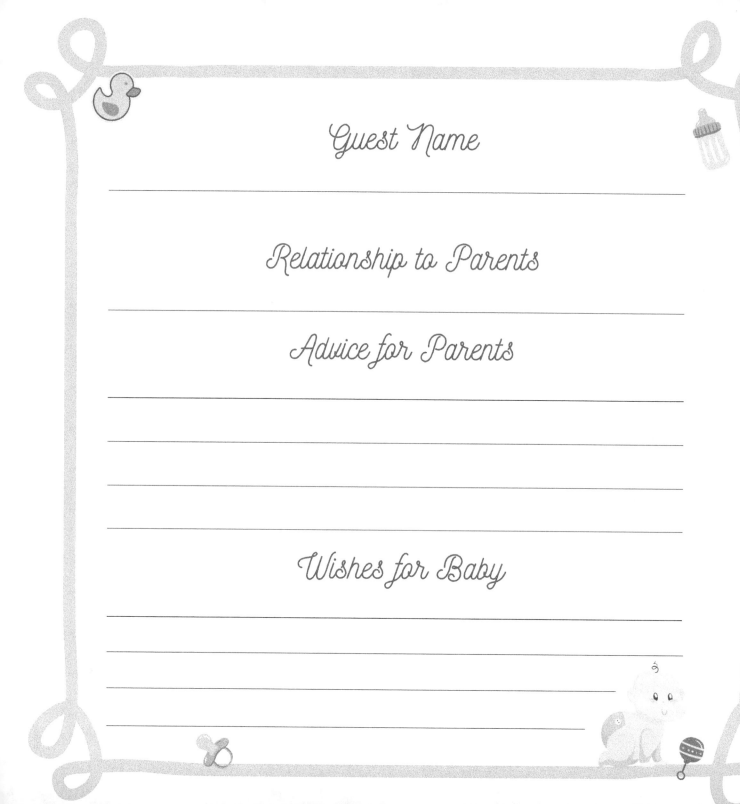

Guest Name

Relationship to Parents

Advice for Parents

Wishes for Baby

Guest Name

Relationship to Parents

Advice for Parents

Wishes for Baby

Guest Name

Relationship to Parents

Advice for Parents

Wishes for Baby

Guest Name

Relationship to Parents

Advice for Parents

Wishes for Baby

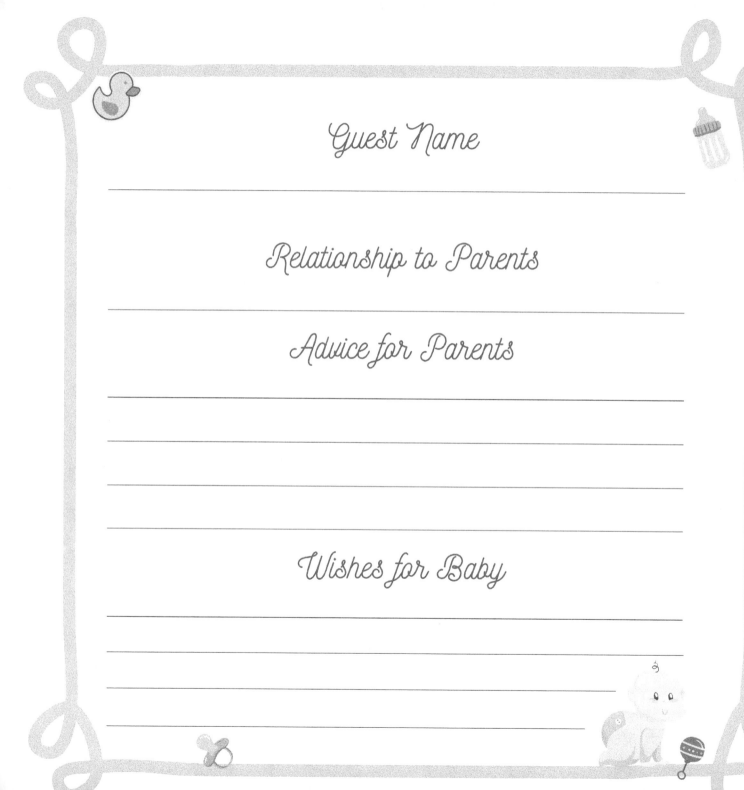

Guest Name

Relationship to Parents

Advice for Parents

Wishes for Baby

Guest Name

Relationship to Parents

Advice for Parents

Wishes for Baby

Guest Name

Relationship to Parents

Advice for Parents

Wishes for Baby

Guest Name

Relationship to Parents

Advice for Parents

Wishes for Baby

Guest Name

Relationship to Parents

Advice for Parents

Wishes for Baby

Guest Name

Relationship to Parents

Advice for Parents

Wishes for Baby

Guest Name

Relationship to Parents

Advice for Parents

Wishes for Baby

Guest Name

Relationship to Parents

Advice for Parents

Wishes for Baby

Guest Name

Relationship to Parents

Advice for Parents

Wishes for Baby

Guest Name

Relationship to Parents

Advice for Parents

Wishes for Baby

Guest Name

Relationship to Parents

Advice for Parents

Wishes for Baby

Guest Name

_____

Relationship to Parents

_____

Advice for Parents

_____

_____

_____

_____

Wishes for Baby

_____

_____

_____

Guest Name

Relationship to Parents

Advice for Parents

Wishes for Baby

Guest Name

Relationship to Parents

Advice for Parents

Wishes for Baby

Guest Name

Relationship to Parents

Advice for Parents

Wishes for Baby

Notes / Photos

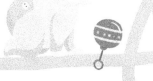

Notes / Photos

Notes / Photos

Notes / Photos

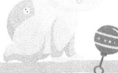

Notes / Photos

Notes / Photos

Notes / Photos

Notes / Photos

Gift Log

Name/Email/Phone   **Gift**

Gift Log

Name/Email/Phone	Gift

Gift Log

Name/Email/Phone   **Gift**

Gift Log

Name/Email/Phone

Gift

Gift Log

Name/Email/Phone

Gift

Gift Log

Name/Email/Phone   **Gift**

Gift Log

Name/Email/Phone	Gift

Gift Log

Name/Email/Phone **Gift**

Gift Log

Name/Email/Phone   **Gift**

Gift Log

Name/Email/Phone	Gift

Printed in the USA
CPSIA information can be obtained
at www.ICGtesting.com
LVHW080838211023
761653LV00004B/149